Published By Robert Corbin

@ Peter Chute

Dirty Sex: Collection of Filthy Taboo Sex & Naughty Romance Erotic Sex Short Stories for Adults

All Right RESERVED

ISBN 978-87-94477-83-3

TABLE OF CONTENTS

Chapter 1 1

40 Sex Positions For Going Deeper 1

Chapter 2 22

Knowing Her Erogenous Zones.......................... 22

Chapter 3 29

Understanding Women 29

Chapter 4 37

Importance Of Sex Education For Boys 37

Chapter 5 47

Our Bodies - Understanding The Male Reproductive System 47

Chapter 6 68

What To Teach Your Teen Girls About Sex And Relationships. 68

Chapter 7 80

Understanding Oral Sex...................................... 80

Chapter 8 87

Things To Avoid When Trying To Get Her Wet 87

Chapter 9 91

Exploring Different Types Of Love 91

Chapter 10 96

The Subtleties Of Anatomy And Physiology On Love, Sex, And Contraception 96

Chapter 11 101

How To Arouse A Woman 101

Chapter 12 112

Controlling Men 112

Chapter 13 126

Building Healthy Relationships 126

Chapter 14 141

My Professional Advice To Teenage Girls On Love And Relationships. 141

Chapter 1

40 Sex Positions for Going Deeper

1. Missionary with a Pillow:

This position involves the classic missionary stance but with a subtle modification. By placing a pillow beneath the woman's hips, you create a slight elevation. This not only enhances comfort but also allows for a deeper angle of penetration, intensifying the experience for both partners.

2. Doggy Style:

A timeless favorite, the doggy style position involves the receiving partner positioning themselves on all fours while the penetrating partner enters from behind. This alignment naturally allows for deeper penetration, offering a more intense and intimate connection.

3. Butterfly Position:

In the butterfly position, the woman lies on her back at the edge of a bed or table, and the man stands. This arrangement facilitates a deeper penetration angle, and the elevated position of the woman's hips can lead to heightened sensations and intimacy.

4. Spooning:

Spooning involves both partners lying on their sides facing the same direction, creating a snug fit. In this position, penetration can be deepened, fostering a sense of closeness and emotional connection, making it an ideal choice for those seeking both physical and emotional intimacy.

5. Legs on Shoulders:

With the woman lying on her back, the man lifts her legs onto his shoulders. This adjustment allows for a more direct and deeper angle of penetration, providing a different sensation and potentially intensifying pleasure for both partners.

6. Deep Missionary:

Building on the traditional missionary position, the deep missionary involves the woman placing her legs on the man's shoulders. This slight alteration creates a deeper entry point, offering a more profound experience for both partners.

7. Edge of the Bed:

This variation of the missionary position involves the receiving partner lying on their back at the edge of a bed. The penetrating partner can stand, allowing for a more pronounced angle of penetration. The edge of the bed provides support and a comfortable platform for exploration.

8. Standing Doggy Style:

In this dynamic position, one partner stands while the other bends over a surface. This allows for deep penetration from behind and introduces an element of standing intimacy, providing a unique and potentially exciting experience.

9. Bridge Position:

The bridge position involves the woman arching her back while the man kneels. This creates a pronounced angle, allowing for deeper penetration. The arched position also adds an aesthetic and sensual element to the encounter.

10. Pile Driver:

Offering a more adventurous option, the pile driver position involves the receiving partner lying on their back and raising their legs, while the penetrating partner stands. This position can provide a deeper and more intense experience, requiring communication and comfort between partners.

11. Lap Dance:

The lap dance position introduces an element of playful intimacy. The woman sits on the man's lap, facing him. This position allows for deep penetration and provides an opportunity for visual and tactile connection. The closeness and direct eye contact can enhance the overall experience, making it both physically and emotionally satisfying.

12. Modified Cowgirl:

A variation of the traditional cowgirl position, the modified cowgirl involves the woman leaning back and supporting herself with her hands. This adjustment not only puts her in control but also allows for deeper penetration. The angle created by leaning back can intensify sensations for both partners, making it a versatile and enjoyable option.

13. Froggy Style:

The froggy style position has the receiving partner lying on their stomach, while the penetrating partner enters from behind. This unique alignment offers deep penetration and a different angle of entry, providing a varied and exciting experience for couples looking to explore new sensations.

14. Seated Wheelbarrow:

In the seated wheelbarrow position, the woman sits on the edge of a surface, and the man stands for penetration. This dynamic arrangement allows for a deep angle and a sense of control for both partners. It also provides an opportunity for increased physical connection and experimentation.

15. Deep Reverse Cowgirl:

Building on the classic reverse cowgirl, this variation involves the woman facing away from the man while he sits. The deeper penetration angle in this position can be particularly stimulating for both partners, offering a different perspective and potentially leading to heightened pleasure.

16. Kneeling Wheelbarrow:

In the kneeling wheelbarrow position, the receiving partner kneels, and the penetrating partner holds their hips. This alignment allows for deep access and an intimate connection. The supportive role of the penetrating partner can add an element of trust and closeness to the experience.

17. Deep Side Spoon:

This variation of the spooning position involves both partners lying on their sides facing each other. The deep side spoon allows for increased penetration depth while maintaining the closeness and comfort associated with spooning. The face-to-face position enhances emotional connection during intimate moments.

18. Inverted Missionary:

The inverted missionary position involves the woman lying on her back at the edge of a bed with her head hanging over. This unique angle allows for a different kind of penetration and can be both visually stimulating and physically intense. It's important to prioritize comfort and communication when trying this position.

19. The Amazon:

In the Amazon position, the woman straddles the man facing him and leans back. This position offers deep penetration and allows the woman to control the rhythm and depth of the encounter. The added visual element and the engagement of core muscles can contribute to a satisfying experience.

20. The Om Position:

The Om position involves both partners sitting cross-legged, facing each other, and connecting intimately. This position allows for deep penetration while fostering a sense of emotional closeness. The eye contact and synchronized movements contribute to a unique and intimate experience for couples exploring deeper connections.

21. Elevated Cowgirl:
The woman straddles the man, but instead of being on her knees, she elevates her hips by balancing on her toes. This can create a unique angle for deeper penetration and allows the woman to control the depth and pace.

22. Spread Eagle:
The receiving partner lies on their back with their legs spread wide, while the penetrating partner

kneels or stands between them. This position allows for deep penetration and offers a visual and physical connection.

23. Seated Lotus:
Both partners sit facing each other with legs crossed and wrapped around each other. This position encourages deep penetration and close contact, fostering intimacy and a strong emotional connection.

24. Reverse Wheelbarrow:
Similar to the wheelbarrow, but with the receiving partner facing away. The penetrating partner holds the hips, providing a unique angle for deep penetration and creating a sense of vulnerability and trust.

25. Scissors:

Both partners lie on their sides, facing each other, with one leg intertwined. This position allows for deep penetration and maintains an intimate face-to-face connection.

26. Lifted Missionary:

The receiving partner lies on their back at the edge of a bed, and the penetrating partner stands. By lifting the receiving partner's hips, this position allows for a deeper angle and enhanced access.

27. Deep Glider:

The woman lies on her back on a smooth surface, and the man kneels while holding her hips. The gliding motion can provide a different sensation and allow for deep penetration.

28. Corkscrew:

The receiving partner lies on their back with legs raised and slightly twisted, while the penetrating partner enters from an angle. This can create a twisting sensation and deeper penetration.

29. Suspended Spoon:

The receiving partner lies on their side at the edge of a bed, and the penetrating partner kneels. This suspended position allows for deep penetration and a sense of weightlessness.

30. Sideways Straddle:

The woman straddles the man while both are lying on their sides, facing the same direction. This position allows for deep penetration with a comfortable side-by-side connection.

31. Deep Squat:

The woman squats over the man while he lies on his back. This position provides a deep angle of penetration and engages the lower body muscles, offering a different physical experience.

32. The Lusty Leg Lift:

The woman lies on her back, and the man lifts one of her legs, creating a deeper angle for penetration. This position allows for a mix of control and intimacy.

33. Bridge of Bliss:

The receiving partner arches their back with hands and feet on the bed, while the penetrating partner kneels. This position allows for deep penetration with a visually stimulating arch.

34. Straddle and Squeeze:

The receiving partner straddles the man facing forward and squeezes her thighs together. This can enhance tightness and provide a unique sensation during deep penetration.

35. The Diamond:

The woman sits on the bed with her legs forming a diamond shape, and the man kneels between them. This position allows for deep penetration and a close connection.

36. Pillow Prop:

The receiving partner places a pillow under their hips during missionary. This simple adjustment can create a more comfortable angle for deep penetration.

37. The Intimate Embrace:

Both partners sit facing each other, legs wrapped around each other. This close, intimate position allows for deep penetration and fosters emotional connection.

38. The Catapult:

The receiving partner lies on their stomach, and the penetrating partner straddles their hips. This position allows for deep penetration with a playful and dynamic element.

39. The Seated Split:

The woman sits on a surface with legs spread wide, and the man kneels or stands between them. This position can provide a deep and intimate connection.

40. Twisted Pleasure:
Both partners lie on their sides facing each other but with their bodies slightly twisted. This position allows for deep penetration and maintains eye contact for a more intimate experience.

In the journey of love, sex, and birth control, it is crucial to begin with a solid foundation of understanding and responsibility. This chapter aims to set the stage by exploring the interconnected themes of love and sex while emphasizing the significance of making responsible choices.

Love: A Powerful Force

Love is a universal language that transcends boundaries and connects individuals on a profound level. It comes in various forms, from romantic love to familial bonds and friendships. Understanding the complexity of love is essential as it forms the backdrop for relationships that may involve intimacy and sexual connections.

Sex: A Natural Expression

Sexuality is an inherent part of the human experience. It's important to recognize the diverse ways people express their sexuality. Whether through emotional connections or physical intimacy, understanding and respecting these differences contributes to fostering healthier relationships.

The Intersection: Love and Sex

When love and sex intertwine, it creates a unique dynamic that requires careful navigation. Exploring one's desires and boundaries, as well as communicating openly with partners, fosters a deeper connection. Building a foundation of trust and respect within a relationship becomes paramount for the well-being of both individuals involved.

Responsible Choices:

The Key to Healthy Relationships

Responsible decision-making is the cornerstone of maintaining healthy relationships. This extends beyond the emotional realm to encompass physical well-being, emphasizing the importance of birth control.

Acknowledging the potential consequences of sexual activity and taking steps to prevent unintended pregnancies requires careful consideration.

Birth Control: Empowering Choices

Understanding the various methods of birth control empowers individuals to make informed decisions about their reproductive health. From contraceptives to family planning, the chapter delves into the options available, highlighting their effectiveness and potential impact on relationship dynamics.

Communication: A Vital Tool

Effective communication plays a pivotal role in navigating the complexities of love, sex, and birth control. Open and honest conversations between partners foster trust and create an environment where both individuals feel comfortable expressing their needs and concerns.

Educating Yourself and Others

In the journey of love, sex, and birth control, continuous learning is crucial. The chapter encourages readers to seek reliable information, stay informed about reproductive health, and share knowledge with their partners.

Education has become a tool for empowerment, allowing individuals to make choices that align with their values and goals.

In conclusion, setting the stage for love, sex, and responsible choices involves understanding the intricate dance between these elements. Love and sex are beautiful expressions of human connection, and when approached with responsibility, they contribute to the development of fulfilling and respectful relationships.

This chapter serves as a guide, encouraging readers to explore these themes with mindfulness and make choices that align with their values and well-being.

Chapter 2

KNOWING HER EROGENOUS ZONES

Erogenous zones are areas of the body that are particularly sensitive to sexual stimulation and can contribute to sexual arousal and pleasure. Keep in mind that the sensitivity of erogenous zones can vary from person to person, and what is pleasurable for one individual may not be the same for another. Here are some common erogenous zones in women:

- **Neck and Ears:** Kissing, nibbling, or gently blowing on the neck and ears can be highly arousing for some women. These areas are sensitive to touch and can create pleasurable sensations.
- **Lips:** Kissing passionately is a fundamental part of sexual arousal for many people. The

lips are highly sensitive and can convey desire and connection.

- **Lower Back and Buttocks:** These areas can be erotic zones for some women. Massaging or caressing the lower back and buttocks can be pleasurable.
- **Lower Abdomen:** Gently touching and kissing the lower abdomen can be a source of arousal. It's an area that's often overlooked but can be quite sensitive.
- **G-Spot:** As mentioned earlier, the G-spot, located on the anterior vaginal wall, is believed by some to be a highly sensitive and pleasurable area when stimulated.
- **Feet:** Some people have sensitive feet, and foot massages or gentle foot caresses can be arousing for them.
- **Back of the Knees:** The back of the knees is a less common but still sensitive erogenous

zone for some women. Lightly kissing or touching this area can be arousing.
- It's important to remember that individual preferences and sensitivity to these zones can vary greatly.
- **Clitoris:** The clitoris is often considered the most sensitive and important erogenous zone in women. It is located at the top of the vulva, under the clitoral hood. Stimulation of the clitoris can lead to intense sexual pleasure and is a key factor in achieving orgasm for many women.
- **Breasts and Nipples:** Many women find that their breasts and nipples are highly sensitive. Gentle caresses, kisses, and nipple stimulation can be arousing for some. However, sensitivity varies, and not all women enjoy this type of stimulation.
- **Inner Thighs:** The inner thighs are a sensitive area that can be erotically stimulating when

touched or kissed. Lightly teasing and caressing this area can build anticipation and arousal.

Knowing Her Non-erogenous zones
Neck

The neck is an area rich in sensitive skin and nerve endings.

Gentle kisses, nibbles, or light strokes on the neck can create a tingling sensation, adding a layer of intimacy and excitement.

Shoulders

Shoulders hold tension and stress and can benefit greatly from a relaxing massage. A soothing shoulder massage not only eases physical stress but also communicates care and comfort, fostering a sense of relaxation.

Arms and Hands

The arms and hands are areas where a soft touch can convey care and affection.

A simple hand massage or gentle caresses on the arms can be a non-verbal expression of love and connection.

Back

The back, especially along the spine, is a pathway to relaxation.

A soothing back rub can release physical tension, creating a tranquil atmosphere and enhancing a sense of closeness.

Legs

The legs, often overlooked, can be a source of sensory pleasure.

Gentle caresses or massages, particularly around the calves and thighs, can offer surprising relaxation and contribute to a holistic physical connection.

Feet

The feet are rich in nerve endings, making them a potential source of pleasure.

A foot massage, with attention to pressure points, not only provides relaxation but also establishes a sense of care and connection.

Engaging with these non-erogenous zones involves recognizing the sensitivity and potential pleasure they offer. Each area provides an opportunity for shared moments of intimacy, whether through massages, gentle touches, or simple acts of affection. While erogenous zones contribute to arousal, the exploration of non-erogenous areas enhances the overall experience of physical connection and emotional closeness.

Chapter 3

Understanding Women

Finding a common language with the woman you love is not easy. Most often than not, a relationship is broken because of these simple misunderstandings. You may have been together for years, yet one could not find the exact formula to truly master interaction with a woman. It is because men and woman are different in so many things.

Hence, if you want a relationship to last, it's not enough to let fate determines everything for you. Unless you get out of the box and make an extra effort to understand a woman's nature, you will never reap the benefits of truly understanding her and be truly understood in return. Only then can you expect a long-lasting relationship with the woman in your life.

Want to have a better and lasting relationship? If you do, then you must know how to treat a woman. Every woman is a "Queen" in her own right and sense. As such, you can give her your best shot through any or all of the following:

Treat A Woman Like a Queen, Not a Bitch!

She doesn't need to be a queen to all, but if you give her the same honor and respect you would grant to a queen, she would never feel in competition with other women for your love.

A woman wants a man she can respect, honor, and treat like the king he is. Mutual respect is an all-or-nothing-proposition for a woman that once she loses respect in you, all bets are off. She may not be equal to your mother, but bestowing her same respect proves you're worthy of her love.

When a woman is made to feel that she's disrespected, the relationship is likely to end sooner than later. Hence; even when you're disappointed or angry, respect should be observed.

Show Her Your Affection

To others, saying "I love you may not be that simple nor easy." There are some people who believe that telling someone this phrase paves the way to a vulnerability that would end up being hurt. Women though deserve to be made aware of your love. If you can't tell her that, you might as well leave her alone. It could be that your feeling towards her is not that great to break your pride. Simply put, you don't love her that much!

How a woman treats you depend on how you are treating her. Once you mistreat her, you are opening the door and give the next guy an opportunity to take her away.

A woman needs a man who can show her kindness, empathy, compassion, patience, and understanding.

Every little thing matters to her like saying "Thank you", "I love you," or "I appreciate you and I wouldn't have made it this far without you!"

Give Her Your Time

Women equate time with love and affection. Don't let her beg for your attention. She believes that you love her enough to share most of your free time with her.

She Wants to be Highly-Valued and Appreciated

A woman would do everything for the man she loves but in return, she expects the same from him. She would spend time in the kitchen just to prepare something for him or she would spend long hours in a spa or beauty salon so the man of her dreams can appreciate her appearance.

Women thrive on positive feedbacks, especially from their partner. To be highly-valued and appreciated reinforces a positive sense of self-worth. Moreover, there is a precious moment of contact when we are recognized and validated.

She Wants a Man With Integrity

Women like to have a relationship with a man who does things the way they say they will and don't make promises they can't afford to keep. Because a woman has an inherent knack to see through you, she can easily detect dishonesty. She knows when you choose to tell her lies even when she doesn't say so. She may love to hear your flatteries but it doesn't mean she believes them.

She also appreciates consistency both in your actions and words. When she notices some discrepancies on these two, she never voiced them out but that surely make a crack on your relationship. For her, words are never enough.

When a woman commits in a relationship, she relies completely on your words. Stability and protection are common expectations knowing she can depend on you to pull her through when the world chooses to turn against her. She wants a man she can respect and honor as she expects to be treated fairly. If you prove to be the man of her dreams, she is willing to face all odds with you even if it means leaving her own family and friend just to be with you.

However, don't make the mistake of thinking that women are dependent on you economically. Smart, independent women can stand on their own and are more interested in a man with principles than in your pocket or bank account.

Don't try impressing her with money as she is more interested in your values and attitudes especially when they are significant to her life. They want to know if you can be a liability or an asset to their achievements.

On top of everything, a woman of faith always puts God above all else and she expects you to respect it.

Realize the Difference in Communication Channel

Men communicate using logic but women on their emotions. Failing to understand this leads to many troubles and usually ends up in a battle of words that ruins a relationship that has been built up through the years. Conflicts can easily arise at any stage of the relationship - from seduction and until the developing stage of the relationship.

In the seduction stage, many guys failed to capture the heart of the women they desire because they want to impress the woman with their intellect and tried to tap into her logical reasoning. A woman may be smart to understand it but it doesn't touch her heart. Women are in search of emotions and it is the passion with which the man speaks about ideas that impress her and not the logic it bears.

Women Longs for Connection

During those precious moments when a woman is seen and appreciated, there's a spontaneous connection that may arise and a woman can be open to that connection. Feeling appreciated strengthens the bond in a relationship between the two people. It helps satisfy her longing for healthy attachment.

CHAPTER 4

Importance of Sex Education for Boys

Let's first discuss what sex education is in reality. Even though we will undoubtedly address the mechanics of sex, it's not just about that. Understanding your body, your feelings, and your relationships are important.

It's about gaining the skills to successfully communicate, set limits, and make decisions that will keep you safe and in good health.

Now, some individuals could believe that girls should only receive sex education. After all, it's usually women that become pregnant. Wrong. Boys, understanding your bodies and your relationships is just as important to you as it is to girls. This is why:

It helps you make informed decisions.

You may choose what you want to do (and what you don't want to do) better when you are aware of the dangers and negative effects associated with various sexual actions.

With this information, you'll be able to safeguard your partner and yourself from unintended pregnancies, STIs, and other health hazards.

It teaches you about consent and respect.
Sexual relationships should always be based on mutual respect and consent. By learning about what consent means and how to communicate effectively, you'll be better equipped to have healthy, positive relationships with others.

It empowers you to take control of your own health.
Sex education isn't just about sex – it's also about understanding your body and how to take care of it.

By learning about hygiene, contraception, and other aspects of sexual health, you'll be able to stay healthy and happy throughout your life.

It helps you build healthy relationships.
Relationships are about more than just sex — they're about communication, trust, and respect. By learning how to communicate effectively and set boundaries, you'll be better equipped to have positive relationships with friends, family, and romantic partners.

It promotes gender and LGBTQ+ equality.
Sex education isn't just for straight, cisgender people. By learning about different gender identities and sexual orientations, you'll be able to be an ally to your friends who may identify differently than you.

You'll be able to challenge harmful stereotypes and stand up against bullying and discrimination.

So, boys, are you starting to see why sex education is so important? It's not just about learning how to put on a condom (although we'll definitely cover that too). It's about understanding your body, your emotions, and your relationships. It's about empowering you to make informed decisions and stay healthy and happy. It's about promoting equality and respect for all people, regardless of their gender or sexual orientation.

So let's dive in and explore this awesome world of sex education together!

Goals of the Book

Okay, let's get into the goals of this book! But first, let me ask you a question: have you ever played a sport without knowing the rules or the goal?

It's difficult to play a game when you don't know what you're attempting to accomplish. The same is true for sexual education. That is why we will discuss the book's objectives.

Our initial goal is to assist you in understanding your body. That's right, we're talking about your entire body, from your head to your toes (and everything in between). We'll go over what each part is for, how it looks, and how it operates.

"Why do I need to know this?" you may wonder. So, if you understand what's going on down there, you'll be better able to care for yourself and communicate with others about what feels good and what doesn't.

Our second purpose is to assist you in comprehending your emotions. Sex is about more than simply physical pleasure, believe it or not. It's also about feelings, such as love, attraction, and want. We'll go over how to recognize and express your emotions in a healthy manner.

You will be able to create stronger and more rewarding relationships with people once you understand your emotions.

Our third purpose is to assist you in better understanding your relationships. Even for adults, relationships can be challenging.

You may, however, develop healthy connections with friends, family, and love partners by learning about communication, respect, and limits.

We'll also discuss consent: what it is, how to obtain it, and how to offer it. You will be able to have positive and respectful sexual experiences if you understand consent.

Our fourth purpose is to assist you in comprehending the world around you. The world is a huge place with a lot of various kinds of individuals. We'll discuss diversity, which includes diverse genders, sexual orientations, and cultures.

You will be able to form meaningful connections with people who are different from you if you appreciate and respect diversity.

Our fifth and last goal is to make sex education enjoyable and interesting! Let's face it: discussing sex might be unpleasant or uncomfortable at first.

But it doesn't have to be that way! We'll utilize delightful and engaging exercises, games, and real-life examples to make learning about sex education enjoyable and engaging.

So, those are the goals of this book: to help you understand your body, emotions, relationships, and the world around you, as well as to make sex education enjoyable! By the end of this book, you will have a solid foundation of knowledge and abilities to make informed decisions and build healthy relationships. Are you ready to get in and begin learning? Let's get started!

How to Use this Book

Welcome to the section on how to use this book! You might be thinking, "I know how to read a book.

Why do I need instructions on how to use it?" Well, this book is a little different from your average novel or school textbook.

We want to make sure you get the most out of it and have fun while you're learning. So, let's go over some tips on how to use this book effectively.

Tip 1: Read it with an open mind

The first thing you should do when using this book is to approach it with an open mind. You might hear things you've never heard before, or things that challenge your existing beliefs or ideas.

That's okay! The point of sex education is to learn and grow, so keep an open mind and be willing to learn new things.

Tip 2: Take breaks

Learning about sex education can be a lot to take in, so don't be afraid to take breaks. You don't have to read the whole book in one sitting. Take a break when you need to and come back to it when you're ready. Maybe even grab a snack or go for a walk – it's all about finding what works for you.

Tip 3: Use the interactive features

We've included plenty of interactive features throughout the book, like quizzes, games, and thought-provoking questions.

Don't skip over these – they're designed to help you engage with the material and make learning fun. Plus, they'll help you remember the information better.

Tip 4: Talk to someone

Sex education can be a sensitive topic, and you might have questions or concerns that you don't feel comfortable discussing with your parents or guardians. That's okay! You can talk to a trusted friend, teacher, or healthcare provider. They can help answer your questions and provide support.

Tip 5: Take action

Sex education isn't just about learning – it's about taking action. Use what you've learned to make informed decisions about your body and your relationships.

Speak up when something doesn't feel right or when you're not sure what to do. Remember that you have the right to make your own choices and set your own boundaries.

So, there you have it – some tips on how to use this book effectively. Keep an open mind, take breaks, use the interactive features, talk to someone, and take action. By following these tips, you'll be well on your way to becoming a sexually informed young boy!

CHAPTER 5

Our Bodies - Understanding the Male Reproductive System

In this chapter, we're going to explore one of the most fundamental aspects of being a boy: understanding your body and the incredible changes it goes through during puberty.

Getting to Know Your Body

Imagine your body as a complex machine with various parts that work together to keep you healthy and growing.

Just like a car engine or a computer, it's essential to understand how everything works.

So, let's start by taking a closer look at the male reproductive system.

The Male Reproductive System

Meet the Star of the Show: Testicles

Your testicles are like the engine of this machine. They may be small, but they have a very important job.

They produce sperm, which are tiny cells that can fertilize an egg to create a baby.

But here's the twist: you won't be able to make babies until you're older. For now, your testicles are just getting ready for the future.

The Tubular Connection: Vas Deferens

The vas deferens is like the highway that carries sperm from your testicles to your urethra. It's a small tube, but it plays a big role when you grow up.

Seminal Vesicles and Prostate Gland: The Helpers

These are the supporting actors in the male reproductive system. They produce fluids that mix with sperm to create semen.

Semen is what comes out of your body during ejaculation, but that's something we'll talk about when you're a bit older.

Testosterone - The Hormone Powerhouse

Now, let's talk hormones. Hormones are like messengers that tell your body what to do.

In your case, testosterone is the big boss. It's responsible for many changes during puberty, like making your voice deeper, growing facial hair, and increasing muscle mass.

It's also the hormone that gives you those strange, sometimes unexpected feelings – like having a crush on someone.

Puberty Is the Game Changer

Right now, you might not see many of these changes happening yet.

That's because puberty, the magical time when these changes occur, usually starts a bit later, around age 12 or 13.

But it's essential to understand what's coming, so you're ready for the adventure of growing up.

Summary

So, here's what you've learned in this chapter:

- Your body is like a well-engineered machine.
- The male reproductive system includes the testicles, vas deferens, seminal vesicles, and the prostate gland.
- Hormones like testosterone are responsible for the changes you'll experience during puberty.
- Puberty is the amazing journey that's just around the corner.

Now that you've got a basic understanding of your male reproductive system, you're better prepared for the exciting changes that lie ahead.

The Basics of Anatomy

Welcome back to our journey of understanding your amazing body!

We are going to keep things simple as we explore the basics of anatomy. Don't worry; we're here to make it fun and easy to grasp.

Let's Get Started

Think of your body as a fantastic puzzle with all the pieces working together to make you who you are.

To solve this puzzle, we need to understand some of the essential parts that make up your body.

The Head - Your Command Center

Your head is like the command center of your body.

It's where your brain lives, and it's responsible for everything you do – from thinking about math problems to daydreaming about your favorite video game.

Your head also houses your senses, like your eyes that see, your ears that hear, and your nose that smells.

The Trunk - Your Strong Core

The trunk of your body is everything from your neck to your hips.

Inside this area, you'll find your heart, lungs, stomach, and other important organs.

Your heart pumps blood, your lungs help you breathe, and your stomach helps digest the yummy food you eat.

The Arms and Hands - Your Handy Helpers

Your arms and hands are like your trusty tools.

You use them for all sorts of things, like playing sports, drawing, and giving high-fives.

They're connected to your body by your shoulders, which allow your arms to move in different directions.

The Legs and Feet - Your Mobile Base

Your legs and feet are like the wheels on a bike. They help you get from one place to another.

Your legs are strong and can carry you on adventures, while your feet keep you steady on the ground.

Bones and Muscles - The Power Duo

Inside your body, you have a fantastic team of bones and muscles.

Bones give your body structure, like the frame of a building, while muscles help you move.

When you want to run, jump, or dance, it's your muscles that do the heavy lifting.

Skin - Your Protective Armor

Your skin is like a super cool suit that wraps around your entire body.

It keeps your insides safe from the outside world and helps you feel things through touch.

Remember to take good care of your skin by keeping it clean and protected from the sun.

Summary
- Your body is like a puzzle with different parts.
- Your head is your command center.
- Your trunk houses important organs.

- Your arms, hands, legs, and feet help you do amazing things.
- Bones and muscles are your body's power duo.
- Your skin is your protective armor.

Understanding the basics of your body is like getting to know your best friend – it makes your adventures together even more exciting.

As you grow up, you'll learn more about how each part of your body works. So, stay curious, and keep exploring this incredible puzzle called "you."

The Role of Hormones

Welcome back to our exploration of growing up and understanding your body.

They're like the superheroes inside your body, and we're here to uncover their incredible powers.

Meet Your Hormones

Imagine hormones as tiny messengers that travel through your bloodstream, giving orders to different parts of your body.

They control many of the changes you'll experience during puberty.

Testosterone - The Main Hero

Let's start with the star of the show: testosterone. It's like the captain of your hormone team.

Testosterone is responsible for many of the changes you'll notice as you grow up, like:

- Increasing muscle mass
- Developing your private parts
- Making your voice deeper
- Growing facial and body hair

Testosterone also gives you those strange, exciting, and sometimes confusing feelings, like having a crush on someone.

It's all part of growing up, and it's entirely normal.

Estrogen - The Important Guest

Even though you're a boy, your body also produces a small amount of estrogen.

It plays a role in your development too, helping your bones grow strong and maintaining healthy skin.

Other Hormones - The Supportive Sidekicks

Besides testosterone and estrogen, there are other hormones in your body that do important jobs.

For example, insulin helps regulate your blood sugar, and adrenaline gets you ready for action when you're excited or scared.

The Puberty Supercharge

Now, you might be wondering when all these changes will start happening.

Well, it's a bit like waiting for the signal to start a race. Puberty, that magical time, is the signal that kicks everything into high gear.

During puberty, your body starts producing hormones like testosterone at a faster rate.

This surge in hormones is like a superhero transformation, and it leads to all those changes we talked about earlier.

Embracing Change

It's essential to remember that everyone's body changes at its own pace. Some boys may start puberty earlier or later than others.

And that's perfectly okay! The most important thing is to embrace these changes as a part of becoming the amazing person you're meant to be.

Summary

- Hormones are tiny messengers that control many changes in your body.
- Testosterone is the main hero responsible for various puberty changes.

- Estrogen plays a role in your development too.
- Puberty is the magical time when your body goes through significant transformations.
- Understanding hormones is like discovering the secret code of your body's growth. As you continue on this exciting journey, remember that you're not alone in experiencing these changes.

How Our Bodies Change During Puberty

Welcome to the exciting world of puberty!

We'll take a deep dive into the incredible changes your body goes through during this transformative phase of your life.

Puberty is like a rollercoaster ride, and understanding it will help you navigate this thrilling journey.

The Puberty Journey

Puberty is a natural and essential part of growing up. It's the period when your body transforms from a child's body into an adult's body.

Think of it as your body's way of preparing for the amazing adventures that lie ahead in your teenage and adult years.

Puberty typically begins around age 12 or 13, but it can start earlier or later for different people.

Remember, everyone's timeline is unique, so there's no need to compare yourself to others.

Physical Changes

Let's start by exploring some of the physical changes that happen during puberty.

These changes are the most noticeable and can sometimes be surprising, but they're entirely normal and a sign of your body maturing.

Growth Spurt

One of the first things you'll likely notice is a significant growth spurt.

Suddenly, you'll find yourself getting taller, and it might seem like your pants are always too short!

This growth is because of the growth plates in your bones closing as you mature.

Private Parts

Your private parts, or genitals, will also undergo changes. Your testicles will start to grow, and your penis will increase in size.

These changes are perfectly normal and are a sign that your body is getting ready for future developments.

Body Hair

As your body matures, you'll begin to notice hair growing in new places.

This includes facial hair, underarm hair, and even some hair around your private area. It's all part of your body's transformation.

Voice Changes

You may have noticed that your voice is starting to sound different.

Your vocal cords are growing and becoming thicker, which makes your voice deeper.

This is why many boys experience voice "cracking" during puberty.

Acne

As your skin goes through changes, you might also start to deal with acne or pimples.

The increase in oil production can lead to skin breakouts. Proper skincare can help manage this.

Sweat and Body Odor

With puberty comes an increase in sweat production, which can lead to body odor.

This is completely normal, and regular bathing and using deodorant can help you stay fresh.

Emotional Changes

Puberty isn't just about physical changes; it's also a time of emotional growth.

Your brain is developing, and this can lead to new feelings and experiences. Here are some emotional changes you might encounter:

Mood Swings

You may find that your moods are a bit unpredictable. One moment you're happy, and the next, you might feel irritable or sad.

These mood swings are entirely normal and are a result of hormonal changes.

Increased Independence

As you get older, you'll likely want more independence and responsibility. You might have a growing desire to make your own decisions and choices.

Friendships and Relationships

Your friendships may become more important to you during puberty. You might also start to develop romantic feelings for others.

It's okay to have these feelings, and it's a natural part of growing up.

The Role of Hormones in Puberty

Remember the hormones we discussed in the previous chapter, like testosterone?

Well, they play a significant role in all these changes. Hormones are like the conductors of the orchestra, directing your body's transformations.

Hormones and Growth

Testosterone is responsible for many of the physical changes you experience.

It triggers the growth spurt, increases muscle mass, and deepens your voice.

Estrogen, although more commonly associated with females, also plays a role in bone growth and maintaining healthy skin.

Hormones and Emotional Changes

Hormones don't just affect your body; they also influence your emotions.

They can cause mood swings, increased emotional sensitivity, and the development of romantic feelings.

Coping with Puberty

Puberty can be an exciting but sometimes challenging time. Here are some tips to help you navigate this period of change:

Talk About It

Don't be afraid to talk to a trusted adult about what you're experiencing. They've been through it too and can offer guidance and support.

Be Patient

Puberty is a process that takes time. Your body will change at its own pace, so be patient and kind to yourself.

Stay Active

Physical activity can help you feel more comfortable in your changing body. It's also a great way to manage stress and stay healthy.

Maintain Good Hygiene

As you produce more sweat and oil, it's essential to keep up with your hygiene routine.

Regular showers, using deodorant, and keeping your skin clean can help.

Seek Information

Educate yourself about the changes happening to your body.

Understanding what's going on can make the process less intimidating.

Be Kind to Others

Remember that your friends are going through similar changes. Be supportive and understanding of them as well.

CHAPTER 6

WHAT TO TEACH YOUR TEEN GIRLS ABOUT SEX AND RELATIONSHIPS.

Moms continue to be one of the most significant people in children's lives long after they are all grown up. Although mother-daughter relationships often have a reputation for being contentious, especially when the girls are teenagers, your guidance is essential to your girl's development.

Teenage years can be very busy and perplexing for a young girl due to a changing body, academic schedule, and mindset. In addition, many contemporary societies continue to place unreasonably high pressure on girls to act and look a certain way, and it is your responsibility as a mother to guide them toward the proper mindset.

I've put together a useful list of suggestions to take into account when speaking with your teenage daughter.

TEACH HER NOT TO BE AFRAID TO SAY NO.

Teenage girls frequently experience peer pressure to conform, whether it's in the context of school, friendships, or romantic relationships. It's important to let her know it's okay to say no, even though being accommodating increases one's overall charisma.

Naturally, most girls will have heard countless lessons at school about not using drugs, so your main piece of advice shouldn't be that. Emphasize the need for your daughter to feel secure in the tasks she accepts and the importance of standing her ground when necessary.

Whether it's engaging in sexual activity, supporting a friend, or even carrying out a task for a superior. Make sure she understands that it's perfectly fine to refuse and to negotiate a solution.

TEACH HER TO ALWAYS REMAIN CONFIDENT

It seems like girls' self-confidence drops by three times by the time they turn 13 years old. They suddenly don't feel like kids anymore, but they also don't feel fully grown up either. Not only should you encourage your daughter to be herself, but you should also model this behavior for her.

Your daughter needs to know that, in the end, how she carries herself will be remembered more than what she wears or accessorizes. Teenagers initially struggle to accept their uniqueness, which is understandable. In addition to offering her this counsel, be sure to acknowledge her for wise choices.

TEACH HER TO ALWAYS PROTECT HERSELF.

Her life will be full of more chances to practice independence as your little girl gets older. She will desire to attend events, spend time with friends, and go on dates. While all of these advancements are fantastic for her mindset, social skills, and confidence, they also raise the possibility of potential risks.

Of course, you shouldn't lock her in the house all day, but you can give her some pointers on how to defend herself in different circumstances. You should talk to your daughter about situations to avoid and how to get help if the unthinkable occurs, in addition to providing protection in hypothetical intimate situations.

LET HER KNOW IT'S OKAY TO CRY

Modern advertisements, publications, and blogs frequently discuss how to raise a strong woman. Although there aren't many drawbacks to raising a bright, determined, and optimistic girl, it's important to note that part of being strong is acknowledging and overcoming one's own flaws.

For instance, if your teen is incredibly upset, you need to make it clear that coming to you and sobbing it out are both acceptable. Sometimes letting one's emotions out, frequently in the form of tears, is the best way to move past a distressing event. Your daughter needs to know that crying does not indicate weakness.

SEE TO IT SHE'S ACTIVE

Your teen daughter should not only cry when faced with heartbreak, a failing grade, or any other upsetting situation. Your daughter needs to remember to always be proactive after accepting her emotions.

Instead of listening to your daughter complain nonstop about a task, somebody, or a relationship, find out what steps she wants to take next. One of the best pieces of advice for adolescent girls is to always consider solutions rather than problems.

Test failure? Make a tutoring group. Relationship problems? Consult a dependable therapist, or handle the issues yourself. Every issue can be solved; your daughter just needs to take the initiative.

REMIND HER THAT SHE CAN REQUEST ASSISTANCE WHENEVER SHE NEEDS IT.

Focusing on strength and independence while raising your daughter has the drawback of making her feel pressured to find solutions to all of her problems by herself. Many teenage girls may feel like a burden or a weak person when they ask for help, whether it's with a friend issue or a challenging math problem on a test. It's crucial that you let her know that everyone requires assistance at times and that she shouldn't be afraid to express her problems.

Make it clear that you're always there for her and ask her if she needs any help before she has a chance to think about asking to give your teen girl the push she needs!

PLEASE TELL HER "EDUCATION IS CRUCIAL"

Although many teenage girls work hard in the classroom throughout their lives, many more may feel pressured to find love, assist with family responsibilities, or divert their attention while still in adolescence.

Regardless of your own educational background, you need to explain to your daughter the value of a good education in today's society and how it will benefit her future. Make an effort to pique her interest in a particular career field and job by giving her examples of what successful women have done with their degrees.

While happiness cannot be purchased, your daughter will have a greater chance of leading a happy, secure life if she receives a better education.

TEACH HER TO ALWAYS STAND UP FOR HERSELF

In any situation, avoiding pointless conflict and confrontation should always be the aim. However, there are some circumstances in which it is unavoidably necessary to defend yourself, particularly as a teenage girl.

Your daughter may find it intimidating to confront a bully or an unfair teacher, but it's crucial that you let her know that there are some situations where confrontation is more than justified.

Remind her to always maintain her composure and kindness while also being assertive in her statements. Be a role model for your daughter at all times and demonstrate how to resolve conflicts amicably.

SHE NEEDS TO CREATE A BUDGET AND TRY WORKING PART-TIME.

Everyone in this world, with the exception of a small group, requires a source of income in order to survive and thrive in contemporary society. Try out part-time work in high school as one of the best ways to gather experience and various necessary skills to succeed in the career world.

Give your daughter advice on the positions she should apply for and assist her in creating a budget so she can keep track of her spending. By doing this, you'll be encouraging your daughter to take her first steps toward financial independence and setting her up for success as an adult.

TEACH HER TO ALWAYS LOVE HERSELF

Even though this piece of advice is the last, your teenage daughter needs to understand it the most. There's a good chance that she will doubt herself and question her self-worth as she goes through puberty and the subsequent adult years.

Bullies, marital problems, academic difficulties, and physical changes could all be sources of stress. You must constantly emphasize to your daughter that she deserves all of your love and that she must learn to love herself. She must first discover how to accept her flaws and unite with her inner spirit in order to successfully navigate the many difficulties of adolescence.

CHAPTER 7

UNDERSTANDING ORAL SEX

All ages and genders of partners frequently engage in oral sex. This position, also known as fellatio or cunnilingus, includes oral stimulation of a partner's anus or genitalia.

Before sexual contact, foreplay frequently includes oral sex. Oral stimulation is frequently used by couples to warm up or get in the mood for sexual activity, but it can also be used during or after. As a standalone act, this role can also be very enjoyable.

How Does It Function?

A partner and the most comfortable position are necessary for oral sex. One partner stimulates the other's penis, vagina, or anus with their mouth, lips, or tongue. In addition to regular genital contact, oral sex allows you and your spouse another way to enjoy each other's company.

85 percent of sexually active persons ages 18 to 44 report engaging in oral sex with a partner of the opposing sex at least once. Oral pleasure isn't just for heterosexual couples, it should be noted. People might appreciate providing or receiving oral stimulation with their partner in same-sex or mixed-sex partnerships.

Difference Between Fellatio, Oral Sex, and Others

There are numerous names for oral sex, both formal and colloquial. Experts have coined their medical names to describe the many forms of oral stimulation:

Fellatio. Lips, tongue, or teeth stimulation of the penis. Although it frequently involves sucking or licking, it can also require using the throat or teeth.

Cunnilingus. tongue stimulation of the clitoris or vagina. Typically, this entails sucking or licking the area around the vulva.

Anilingus. using the mouth or lips to stimulate the anus.

Although these are the clinical terms, oral sex can also be described by less formal phrases, such as:

Rimming

69

Blow job

Going down

Giving head

The Myths of Oral Sex

Even if oral sex may be a pretty frequent practice, there are certain myths about it:

Myth: Oral sex isn't sex. Many young people and college students, according to studies conducted in the previous several decades on them, do not view oral sex as real sex. Instead, they view it as a delightful, low-risk activity that lets them keep their virginity. Additionally, studies reveal that many teenagers and young people experiment with oral sex before having genital contact.

Oral pleasure is still seen as a sexual act even if it differs significantly from sexual intercourse. Oral sex is a private act that involves genital contact. It carries some of the same risks as sexual activity, but it can also be just as enjoyable.

Myth: Oral sex is completely risk-free. There is still a chance of contracting an STD during oral intercourse even though there is no possibility of becoming pregnant (STD). Although the danger of contracting an STD from oral sex is slightly lower than from genital sex, it still exists. Typical STDs that can be transmitted orally include:

Chlamydia

HIV

Syphilis

Herpes

Gonorrhea

How to Safely Try Oral Sex

All genders are capable of having or receiving oral sex, but it's crucial to make sure that both parties are ok with it.

Ask your lover if you can try oral sex. The first step is to discuss providing each other oral pleasure with your spouse. According to some studies, heterosexual women may be less likely to request sexual gratification from their male partners. The same study, though, also revealed that men desired to engage in oral sex with their spouses more frequently.

Because oral stimulation is such a private act, discuss ways you might enjoy each other. You can start by kissing and touching your lover before progressively utilizing your lips in a way that they find pleasing.

Possible Dangers

The possibility of catching an STD exists during oral intercourse. Use protection, such as a condom or dental dam, if you are having casual oral intercourse. These products can safeguard you and your partner while reducing your risk of contracting an STD.

To prevent further issues, refrain from oral sex if you or your partner have cuts, sores, or ulcers in your mouth, around your genitals, or on your anus. Not all STD symptoms are immediately apparent and might affect fertility and general health.

CHAPTER 8

THINGS TO AVOID WHEN TRYING TO GET HER WET

To make a girl wet, guys sometimes resort to unorthodox methods. Whereas these methods might produce some results with specific individuals, they are better to be avoided, unless recommended by a medic.

Lubricating sprays and gels

There are some lubricating sprays and gels which can provide required moisture, but the results are varied. The sprays usually need to be applied few minutes before the intercourse. This action alone may kill the romance a bit, or in the least, bring down the levels of your excitement, but many couples use this type of alternative.

However, using artificial sprays may come with consequences. Even though they are marketed as water based sprays and gels, they often contain other chemicals, such as triglycerides, glycerol, sorbitol, phenoxyethanol, flavors, mentholthan, etc.

Some girls may experience an allergic reaction to some of the chemicals of lubricating sprays and gels, which is not a pleasant thing in such sensitive areas.

Instead of using any type of external lubrication, perhaps focus on kissing and touching her a bit longer. Explore her sensual and erotic zones and take your time. Give her a chance to get enough stimulation from you to awaken her state of sexual arousal.

Consuming alcohol to get a girl wet

Remember that in most countries the legal age for alcohol consumption is 18. If you provide alcohol to a minor and proceed with sexual advances towards that person, you may have to face horrible consequences in the future.

Alcohol is known to spike reactions in the human body. More often than not heavy alcohol intoxication makes people lose control and do things they normally wouldn't do.

Alcohol does not do anything directly to get her wet, but it helps the muscles and the body to relax.

During an intoxicated state our thoughts, desires and behavior may undergo a significant change. While sometimes a little bit of alcohol may act as a sexual stimulant, too much alcohol may lead to nausea, vomiting, and possibly alcohol poisoning, which may require hospitalization.

Chapter 9

Exploring Different Types of Love

Love, in its myriad forms, is a force that binds individuals and shapes the tapestry of human relationships. Understanding the diverse expressions of love is crucial for building healthy connections. In this chapter, we delve into the various types of love, illuminating the spectrum that extends beyond romantic entanglements.

Romantic Love:

The quintessential depiction of love, romantic love is characterized by passion, intimacy, and commitment. It often serves as the foundation for long-term
 partnerships and marriages. Exploring shared interests, fostering open communication, and

nurturing emotional connections are essential components of building a robust romantic relationship.

Familial Love:

The bonds forged within families are some of the strongest and most enduring. Familial love encompasses unconditional support and is shared between parents and children, siblings, and extended family members. Building healthy familial relationships involves cultivating empathy, resolving conflicts constructively, and appreciating individual differences.

Platonic Love:

Platonic love, devoid of romantic or sexual attraction, thrives on deep emotional connections and mutual understanding. Friendships, typically lasting a lifetime, are grounded in trust, shared experiences, and a genuine appreciation for one another. Cultivating platonic love involves investing time and effort in friendships, celebrating achievements, and offering support during challenging times.

Self-Love:

An often overlooked yet crucial form of love, self-love is the foundation for overall well-being. Building a healthy relationship with oneself involves self-acceptance, self-compassion, and prioritizing personal growth. Practicing self-care, setting boundaries, and acknowledging one's worth contribute to positive and resilient self-love.

Unrequited Love:

Navigating the complex terrain of unrequited love requires resilience and self-awareness. Understanding that love is not always reciprocated, and embracing personal growth through such experiences can lead to valuable insights. Building healthy relationships, even when faced with unrequited love, involves maintaining respect for boundaries and recognizing when it's necessary to move forward.

Altruistic Love:

Altruistic love transcends the personal sphere, extending outward to encompass compassion and empathy for humanity at large. Engaging in acts of kindness, volunteering, and contributing to the community are ways to express altruistic love. Building healthy relationships on this foundation involves fostering a sense of social responsibility and shared values.

Erotic Love:

Exploring the sensual and physical aspects of love is integral to a comprehensive understanding of human connections. Open communication, consent, and mutual respect are paramount in building healthy erotic relationships. Embracing one's desires, while respecting the boundaries of others, contributes to fulfilling and respectful erotic love.

In conclusion, love is a multifaceted gem with various facets that shine uniquely in different relationships. Nurturing healthy connections requires a nuanced understanding of these diverse expressions of love. Whether navigating the complexities of romantic entanglements, celebrating the enduring bonds within families, or fostering Platonic connections, the key lies in cultivating empathy, communication, and mutual respect.

As we explore the vast terrain of love, we lay the foundation for meaningful relationships that enrich our lives in profound ways.

Chapter 10

The Subtleties of Anatomy and Physiology on Love, Sex, and Contraception

Human Orchestra: Anatomy

Intimacy is based on a deep understanding of human anatomy. The human body is a complex symphony of interconnected systems that play a vital role in the dance of love and desire.

Nervous System:

Acting as the conductor of this symphony, the nervous system transmits signals that initiate and regulate intimate responses. From gentle caressing touches to heightened sensations of passion, nerves convey the language of desire.

Endocrine System :

Hormones, the messengers of love, are secreted by the endocrine system. From adrenaline that creates excitement to oxytocin that drives connection, these chemical signals contribute to the emotional tapestry of intimacy.

Reproductive System:

At the heart of the topic of love and contraception is the reproductive system. Understanding the menstrual cycle, ovulation, and fertilization is vital as couples navigate their intimacy and family planning journey.

2. The Dance of Physiology:
How the Body Is Connected

Physiology, the study of how our bodies function, is inextricably intertwined with the dance of intimacy. From arousal to climax, physiological responses shape the intimate experience.

Sexual Response Cycle

The sexual response cycle created by Masters and Johnson consists of the stages of arousal, plateau, orgasm, and resolution. Understanding this cycle gives people the ability to explore and communicate their needs to their partner.

Cardiovascular System :

In moments of passion, blood flow is regulated by the cardiovascular system. Healthy blood flow is not only essential for alertness but also promotes overall well-being and vitality.

Muscular System:

A lover's embrace, and rhythmic movements, are all expressions controlled by the muscular system. Strength, flexibility, and control enhance the physical aspects of intimacy.

2. Communication: The Glue of Intimacy

In the symphony of love, effective communication acts as the glue that binds partners together. Honest and open communication about needs, boundaries, and expectations is the key to a harmonious relationship.

Verbal Communication:

Expressing your feelings, needs, and problems verbally creates a bridge of mutual understanding. Clear communication fosters emotional intimacy by creating a safe space for vulnerability.

Nonverbal Communication:

Subtle clues such as body language, warmth of touch, and The intensity of eye contact convey unspoken emotions. Paying attention to these nonverbal clues increases the depth of your connection.

Empathy and Understanding:

Empathy for your partner's experiences, fears,

and joys creates a deep emotional connection. Understanding each other on a deeper level strengthens your bond and creates a positive environment.

Finally, the chapters covering anatomy and physiology in the context of love, sex, and contraception are a journey into the intricacies of the human body. By demystifying the physical self and by practicing effective communication, couples can navigate a path to intimacy based on understanding, respect, and overall satisfaction.

Chapter 11

HOW TO AROUSE A WOMAN

As a man, if you think women experience arousal the same way you do, you're wrong. Making a woman horny is not something random that you do with little effort. It's an art in itself and only real men can realize this. You might have come across men who brag about themselves and things they can do thinking that technique might make a woman fall for them. You might have also seen men ignoring women, thinking playing hard-to-get will make women wet and horny. But it's all wrong and it only means you need to understand what truly works if you want to arouse a woman. First and foremost, you need to stop seeing women as objects that you can turn on any time you want. A woman should be respected in all ways. She needs to know that she is seen and heard. You need to allow yourself to get vulnerable in front of her. Don't ever let her feel that she's nothing to you. Don't act all bossy. It's a two way thing don't just call her when you're horny or when you just want to satisfy yourself. Making love is a two way thing and the desire should be from both parties.

Understanding Female Arousal

One of the best ways to get your partner in the mood for sex is to be present and engaged.

Giving your partner your full attention before you reach the bedroom, such as putting your phone away and having a meaningful conversation at the dinner table, will do more to get her in the mood than just lighting a few candles. Don't get me wrong because lighting candles is also important.

That being said, setting the mood is also important.

It's advisable for men to engage in a bit of 'choreplay', that is, helping to arrange and tidy the house and do your part when it comes to chores, so that she has more time to relax and practice self-care.

If you think instant dirty talking will help, you need some learning because that's vague. Dirty talking can surely help, but you shouldn't begin with it as your first move. The best way to make a woman feel aroused is by making them feel special. How do you do that? Well, for starters, you show her that you're different from the rest of the men out there. You pay attention to her personality and not her looks. You study her so you can know what she wants and what she doesn't either sexually or not. A woman needs to be heard, cared for, she wants to know you're making an effort.

The forgotten art of seduction

Courting in modern-time means talking about the things that you can do for a woman regardless of your bank account, social status, etc. It's about the little things that mean a lot to a woman.You don't have to wait till you have enough money(even if it's needed). You need to treat her like your friend first, invest time in getting to know her better. Ask her meaningful questions and delve into deep conversations instead of small meaningless talks. The most important aspect of arousal is communication. Talk to your partner about their desires, boundaries, and what they find arousing. Everyone is different, so understanding your partner's preferences is essential.

Think of your partner like a slow-cooker – don't rush things.

To build up to a cozy evening together, set a good vibe all day. You could also Send her sweet and flirty texts Tell her she looks great in her new dress Help out by doing the dishes, giving her time for yoga Share a glass of wine on the couch Create a chill, romantic atmosphere that she'll love.

Make Eye Contact

During foreplay, you'll be enjoying the view of her beautiful body.

Remember to look directly into her face, making lots of eye contact.

Many women find this super attractive as it creates a direct connection. This simple thing can make her feel admired and wanted.

A woman might notice a good-looking man who hits the gym, has fine facial features and knows tons of big words. But he won't be able to make her horny just with physical appearance. A man needs to establish an emotional connection with a woman, otherwise, he won't succeed in turning her on. Allow the woman to express herself, listen to her carefully and reciprocate no matter how long it takes. It's about stimulating a woman's mind instead of her body. Doing this indirectly stimulates her body as it is really hard for a woman to experience arousal without feeling an emotional connection. My point is women have very sensitive sexual organs so if you build a very strong emotional connection with a woman and you're able to make her yearn for you…You're halfway there already because you already have her on chokehold. This is just to say making a woman horny is not all about kissing and touching. A woman can be horny just by seeing you. Then it's left to you to actually work on these areas.

Treat her like she's the only woman you have eyes for

As a man, why would you even treat your woman with little or no respect? And then you just think when she sees you she'll get in the mood? You're definitely getting it wrong. Take care of your woman, be a gentle man?, Flirt with her, but most importantly, be gentle with her. Don't show off your masculinity. Sure, you can mention certain things that you are really proud of, but don't let your achievements be the main topic of discussion. This is a turn off for most women. If you want to make a woman feel aroused, you need to observe her body language and listen to her. Make her feel at ease. This will help you be one step ahead of the game. Remember that nothing beats communication when it comes to pleasing a woman either sexually or not. Communicate with her. Know what she likes and what she doesn't then you can now move to the next step.

How you kiss is important

You should be able to kiss in a very sensual and erotic way. Start slowly and work your way towards a passionate and rough kiss. Use your fingers to run through her hair. Look into her eyes slowly, you can also make her anticipate. I mean you can touch her lips gently with light kissing her, Give her little time to catch her breath and take her by surprise by even nibbling her jaw, and ears. That'll definitely work!

Find Out What She Enjoys

Being a good listener is attractive to women.
Ask her about her preferences and really pay attention to what she says. It helps you understand what she likes.

Before getting started, have a little chat. Ask about her fantasies and share yours. Discussing desires before the action can be a big turn-on.

Talking about sex beforehand is a great way to get each other in the mood.

Foreplay, foreplay and foreplay!

Engaging in sound foreplay is the key to satisfying your woman. You can start with the neck and work your way towards her waist, leaving kisses and hickeys behind. Make sure you go slow because ending the foreplay quickly is going to leave her high and dry. Also explore different ways to stimulate your partner's senses. This can include using scents, soft music, or even different textures to enhance the experience.

Use Your Fingers

Explore manual techniques for intimate pleasure. While attending to your partner's clitoral region, use your hand's palm to apply gentle pressure on the surrounding vulva, enhancing stimulation across the entire clitoral body. Alternatively, softly press just above the pubic mound for external G-spot pressure. If your partner desires vaginal stimulation, consider inserting one or two fingers, experimenting with thrusting, a "come hither" motion, or steady pressure against the front vaginal wall. If your partner is open to it, you can also explore anal play with proper lubrication for a comfortable experience.

Dirty talk for the win

Erotic, sensual dirty talk is how you can make your woman writhe in pleasure and satisfaction. If you're not aware of how you can engage in dirty talk, you can always read erotic books to get an idea. Your woman will definitely love the idea of you whispering the things you'll do to her, in her ear. Discuss and explore each other's fantasies, as long as it's done consensually and respectfully. Always respect your partner's boundaries and be willing to adjust your approach if something doesn't feel right for her. Know when you stop if her energy is low.

Chapter 12

Controlling Men

He could be any woman's ideal man – charming, intelligent, funny, loving, thoughtful, and kind. He seems to be perfect unless he stopped being one!

Everything happens gradually. At first, you thought, he was just too over-protective – almost keeping you at his side most of the time, helping you and being overly-attentive. He wants the best for you so he openly says what's good for you. Then he started dictating. All those friendly tips and suggestions transformed into criticisms and demands pressuring you to follow his orders. What was once his charming way to get what he wants became an open manipulation and his kindness depends on how you take him and all his demands. Your Prince Charming morphed into a controlling Alpha mate who is a control freak.

Men who are controlling don't necessarily have to look like those tough guys on the screen who would bully the lead star. In fact, most of them are the smart-looking and soft-spoken friendly guy next door. He has the ability to fool even the smartest woman prior to hooking her. Only then would he reveal his true nature to her.

They don't need to be a spoiled brat kid with a rich dad at his beck and call. He could be anybody of any background who demands that everything should be his way and he knows exactly how to exert control in his intimate relationship.

A controlling man has a great arsenal of weapons – shaming, blaming, shutting you down, and even isolating you from your own self - to ensure that you follow every command lest you suffer consequences. His initial strategy is brainwashing and this includes isolation from your loved ones – friends and family.

Living with a controlling freak is like living in hell. When self-expression is a big part of a woman's identity, losing it or trying to change her compromises her freedom.

Being in a controlling relationship is a conglomeration of psychological abuses – physical, emotional, mental, and even spiritual which are depriving and demeaning to a woman.

The change in behavior can come slowly like a silent killer or as a sudden blow that can kill with intensity leaving one wondering what made him change overnight. The most difficult part of this kind of relation is relieving the memories and dissecting each part just to know why it happens. Why the sudden change. You would be wondering if you have done something wrong."

Regardless of what you did, things are bound to happen. Controlling men have been like that ever since. It's just that they are good in concealing their real nature to entrap the woman.

You may have noticed the early warnings at the start but you dismissed it in favor of what you thought was a fabulous romance. Before you realize it, it was too late!

So if you have not been in a controlling relationship before, spot the early signs to avoid a traumatic life ahead. Here are some of the controlling signs you might see in your partner.

Controlling Signs to Spot If Your Partner is Someone You Don't Know

Ever been in a hostile-oriented relationship? If ever there is one, being with a controlling partner is the best example one can have.

Being in this kind of relationship always puts you in a struggling position and battle with yourself if not with him. It is all about what he wants and laying aside what you want. This is destructive not only to your relationship but to your life as a person that even if you manage to get out of it alive, you are sure to develop Post Traumatic Stress Disorder (PTSD).

All his decisions, needs, desires, and interests subdued your own that trying to voice out your points could end up in a violent reaction.

Women love to be treated with respect and not controlled by manipulation. As soon as you spot the following signs, make your headway lest you'll be caught in his manipulative trap. At the start of your relationship, draw the lines. Make sure that you have clear boundaries before you commit to someone in a relationship.

He's a Real Bully

It's not that hard to recognize the overt ways of a bully partner especially when he often pushes you around just to get what he wants. There are many ways he can do to express his bully side – like when he yells at you in an attempt to block you from expressing your point of view, but what if your partner is someone who employs more subtle but manipulative ways to control you? Ways that confuse you and leave you feeling embarrassed to challenge him or when you are feeling guilty for any misdeed you did not cause are just some of the bullying ways controlling men can use just to make you submissive to his will.

Bullying is his primary weapon as he refused to acknowledge whatever ideas or points you are presenting. If you are not apt to his bullying method, he can resort to many other tactics like pouting, making you feel you're on the wrong side, or even display a sullen look just so you will give in. Over time, you will learn to go along in all his decisions which unfortunately aid him in tightening the reins on you.

Emotional bullying does not require physical threats. One can bully a partner by simply causing them misery through any of the following:

- Controlling the purse strings
- Throwing tantrums
- Calling them names
- Withholding love or sex
- Employing the cold-shoulder treatment

There are many motivations for bullying as they tried to cover up their own feeling of low-esteem and inadequacies by trying to put down their partner. Bullies are typically egocentric and narcissistic and are uncaring of the impact of their behavior on others.

He's an Egoistic Critic

When before, he seems to admire every part of you, as you become more comfortable in his presence, he will suddenly be criticizing you in almost everything. If he doesn't like your make up or dress, he will bluntly tell you so or make a joke of it, disregarding your feeling. The same thing when you achieve something that will put him uneasy.

It's a controlling man's goal to force you into mental submission so he can easily manipulate you to do just what he wants. He will make you believe that you are nothing without him. Giving out ultimatums, deceptions, and telling you lies are all part of a controlling man's ability to subject you completely under his power.

When giving in to his manipulation, you will begin to doubt your own ability to make sound judgments. All this will deflate your self-esteem and you begin to lose your self-confidence. What's worst, as he has his clout over you, you believe that everything he's doing is just right because he cares for you? All those manipulative acts are taking a toll on you.

He is Abusive

As thing go deeper and while you are isolated from people who would be running to your rescue, he would start calling you names, show disrespect, and placing all the blame on you. But still, he will lead you to believe that everything is your fault and was just trying to correct your mistakes. You will be subjected to sexual abuse and domestic violence and be treated inferior, making you a prisoner in your own body.

He now owns you and yet treated you without value. Over time, this can leave you with a feeling of being unloved and always lacking.

With subtle comments or overt criticism, he is putting a wedge between you and those people you care for and who love you in return, like your families and best friend as your controlling partner wants you to depend only on him. He wants you to be fully dependent on him in all his demands and decisions so that he can have your full attention for his needs.

For him, you are just something he possesses, something he owns and someone who should give in to all his whims and schemes. Your love for him is just a tool that he can use against you or manipulate you. He is aware of how much you crave for his love and attention and he is taking advantage of this. He expects you to be there at his beck and call.

He is too Possessive

A possessive partner at the start of your relationship is something you may find appealing as you consider it a display of his attention and love for you. But over time, his possessiveness becomes twisted and dark – being constantly suspicious of your actions and motives. Even the most innocent interaction with someone on the opposite sex is seen as malicious flirting. Being paranoid about losing his claws on you, your controlling partner tends to be suspicious of anyone which is also one of the reasons why he had to isolate you away from your family and friends.

You're always subject to a constant check like where did you go? Who are you calling? Who is that guy? Why do you have to buy this and that? Although he bombarded you with questions, he didn't really care about your answers.

A controlling man can be relentless in his arguments. They can tighten the screw of guilt until you give in because you lose the energy to put up with him and this could happen all the time.

His jealousy and over-protective acts seem helpful at first. Women easily get trapped in this display of affection but when the partner takes too much control in your relationship, it may start to cripple your self-esteem and self-worth. The more dependent you become; the more that he will take over the whole control of your life. It may be less work for you at the start of the relationship only to find out later that you have very little power if none at all.

They are Emotional Manipulators

When you are too sweet and caring and sensitive to your partner's emotion, it's the other way around with a controlling man. He has mastered the art of making you feel guilty for any fault you have never committed. He is good in locating your Achilles heel and play with your emotions like the fool you are.

Controlling men have their masterful ways of letting you believe that you are at fault when something went wrong and that you can only correct this by following his rules and guidelines.

It's common and natural to ask for permission on what to wear, when to leave the house, when to speak, or when to shut up. He is the master of your life for he believes you are his property and he owns you and everything about you. This is the reason why he isolates you from others – especially from your family and friends.

Because you are alone, you are trapped – nowhere to go and no one to help you. He is free to randomly yell at you to create a hostile environment which he entirely controls. For him, you are someone he doesn't value nor appreciate aside from what you can do for him, but he will lead you to believe that he loves you and what he's doing with your life is for your own good. Any resistance from your part could lead to severe physical discipline and abuse.

Ultimately, controlling men's objective is to break your spirit and destroy your will to fight for yourself. This will soon cause you to lose your self-confidence and belief in your ability. Suffering from Post-Traumatic Stress Disorder is one thing you will acquire eventually.

CHAPTER 13

Building Healthy Relationships

As you become older, you'll develop a variety of relationships with the people around you. You'll have friends, family, instructors, coaches, and possibly a crush or two. However, not all relationships are equal. Some can be beneficial and healthy, while others might be toxic and detrimental.

So, what constitutes a healthy relationship? Here are a few things to remember:

Communication:

Good communication is the foundation of any healthy relationship. That means listening to each other, speaking honestly and respectfully, and working through problems together.

Respect:

You should always treat others with respect, no matter who they are or what they've done. That means listening to their opinions, valuing their feelings, and treating them the way you'd like to be treated.

Trust: Trust is essential in any relationship. You need to be able to rely on each other, keep promises, and respect each other's privacy.

Boundaries:

It's important to set boundaries in any relationship, whether it's with a friend, family member, or romantic partner. That means knowing your limits and expressing them clearly, and respecting other people's boundaries as well.

Fun: Healthy relationships are also enjoyable and fun! You should be able to have a good time with the people in your life, whether you're playing sports, watching movies, or just hanging out.

But how do you actually build healthy relationships? Here are a few tips:

Be yourself:

The best relationships are built on honesty and authenticity. Be true to yourself, and you'll attract people who appreciate and respect you for who you are.

Listen: Remember, communication is key! Listen to what others have to say, and show that you care about their thoughts and feelings.

Practice empathy:

Try to put yourself in other people's shoes and understand their perspective. This can help you build stronger connections and avoid misunderstandings.

Be open-minded:

Everyone is different, and that's what makes the world interesting! Keep an open mind and be willing to learn from others, even if they're very different from you.

Have fun: Remember, healthy relationships are also enjoyable! Don't forget to have fun and make positive memories with the people in your life.

By building healthy relationships, you'll not only create a positive and supportive environment for yourself, but also make the world a better place. So go out there, be kind, and make some awesome new friends!

Understanding Emotions and Empathy

Have you heard the expression "put yourself in someone else's shoes"?

It's a term that signifies attempting to understand how someone else feels by imagining yourself in their shoes. Understanding and sharing someone else's feelings is what empathy is all about.

It might be difficult to grasp how another person feels, especially if we have never experienced the same situation. But it doesn't mean we can't give it a shot.

Paying attention to how other people react to situations is one method to cultivate empathy.

Someone who is crying, for example, may be sad or distressed. Someone who is smiling and laughing may be joyful or thrilled. We can begin to grasp how someone else is feeling by paying attention to these clues.

Another key aspect of empathy is the ability to demonstrate our concern. This can be giving someone a hug, a nice remark, or simply listening to them when they need to talk. It's not always necessary to tell someone that we're here for them.

But what about our feelings? It's also crucial to recognize and express our own emotions. It's normal to feel angry, depressed, or annoyed at times.

We can express our feelings to someone we trust, such as a parent, teacher, or friend. They could be able to provide assistance and make us feel better.

It's also crucial to understand that everyone's feelings are unique. Just because someone else does not react in the same manner that we do does not make their sentiments any less valid.

Even if we don't entirely comprehend how someone else feels, we can cultivate empathy by being kind and supportive.

Role-playing with a friend or family member is a fun approach to cultivate empathy. You can take turns pretending to be someone else and envisioning how they might react in a given situation.

This can help you develop empathy while also being a pleasant exercise to conduct with someone else.

Remember that empathy is a valuable quality to have in life. It assists us in developing healthy relationships and better understanding the world around us.

So, the next time you talk to someone, put yourself in their shoes and observe how you feel. You might be amazed at how much empathy can teach you and help you grow.

Here's a fun story to help illustrate the concept of empathy:

Tim was a tiny boy who lived once upon a time. One day as Tim was headed to school, he noticed his friend Mike crying on the pavement. Mike had tripped and scraped his knee, which was bleeding.

Tim was concerned for his friend and wanted to make him feel better. He was aware that when he received a scrape or a cut, it hurt a lot and made him miserable.

So Tim sat down next Mike and wrapped his arm around him. He apologized for injuring Mike and said he understood how he was feeling.

Mike looked up at Tim once he had stopped crying. He grinned and thanked him for his friendship. Tim was pleased that he could make Mike feel better.

Tim made it a point from then on to constantly look out for his pals and show empathy when they were down.

He realized how vital it was to attempt to understand how people felt and to offer support and comfort whenever they needed it.

Types of relationships

Have you ever heard the expression "No man is an island"? That's because humans are social beings that enjoy forming connections with others.

We build all types of relationships throughout our lives, from playground friends to family members we see at holiday feasts to the special someone we might meet someday.

Let's start with friends - aren't they the best? Friends are people who share your interests and can make you laugh till you cry. They're the people you turn to when you're down, and they'll always have your back.

But did you realize that it's also crucial to work on your friendships? You must be a good listener, communicate your feelings, and be truthful. Remember that you receive back what you give!

Family is a little different from friends in that you can't actually choose them. Your family loves you and wants what's best for you, even if they can drive you crazy at times. Even if you don't always agree, show them some love and respect.

Then there's romance...we know it's not on your radar right now, but it's still vital to learn about! When you develop feelings for someone special, you may want to spend more time with them and get to know them better.

It is critical to be patient and honest with yourself and with others, as well as to respect their sentiments.

As an example, consider a soccer team. We all have many types of connections in our lives, just like a soccer team.

Family relationships are analogous to team members. Your family members are the ones who will always have your back, just as your teammates do on the field.

They inspire you to achieve your best and cheer you on, just like your family members do for you in whatever you do.

Friendships are analogous to the spectators in the stands. Your friends are the people who come to cheer you on from the sidelines.

They may not be on the field with you, but they are an essential member of your squad.

Romantic relationships are analogous to the coach. A love partner can be someone who supports and inspires you to be the best you can be, much as the coach directs and advises the team.

They may not be on your squad, but they are still significant in your life.

Remember that, just as each player on a soccer team has a certain function to play, each relationship in your life is distinct and valuable in its own right.

Whatever type of relationship it is, it is always necessary to put forth some effort to make it work. You must speak with one another, listen to one another, and demonstrate that you care.

And who knows, you might just make some of your fondest memories with the people with whom you form these relationships!

Consent and boundaries

It's critical to grasp the principles of consent and boundaries in partnerships. Simply said, consent is the act of giving permission, while boundaries are the act of establishing limits.

"But I'm just a kid!" you may be thinking. "Why should I care about consent and boundaries?" The truth is that you have the right to say "yes" or "no" to things that make you uncomfortable, even at a young age. It's also critical to respect other people's rights to say "yes" or "no."

Let us begin with the idea of consent. Everyone participating in an action or situation has given their consent. This could range from playing a game with friends to hugging someone.

anything's not okay to do anything if everyone concerned hasn't agreed to it. For example, it is not acceptable to push your friend to play a game that you have suggested.

It's critical to remember that just because someone doesn't say "no" doesn't imply they agree. It's critical to pay attention to what they say and their body language. If they appear uneasy or reluctant, it's better to inquire if they're okay with what's going on. And if they say "no," you must respect their decision.

Let us now discuss boundaries. Boundaries are the restrictions we place on ourselves in order to feel safe and comfortable. It's okay to say "no" to activities that push your boundaries, even if other people are fine with it.

It's okay to say "no" and propose a different game if someone wants to play a game that makes you uncomfortable.

It is also critical to respect the boundaries of others. If someone says "no" to anything, it's crucial to listen to them and not force them to do it anyhow.

Consider how everyone has a "bubble" surrounding them when thinking about consent and boundaries. This bubble symbolizes our personal space and boundaries.

It is acceptable for individuals to approach our bubble, but it is not acceptable for them to break it without our permission. It's also not right for us to burst someone else's bubble without their permission.

Remember that understanding consent and boundaries is a critical component of developing successful relationships. It is never too early to begin learning about them!

CHAPTER 14

MY PROFESSIONAL ADVICE TO TEENAGE GIRLS ON LOVE AND RELATIONSHIPS.

MAKE SURE YOU SET BOUNDARIES FROM THE START.

Teenagers are always vulnerable, both emotionally and physically. Having boundaries in a relationship can often keep it in balance. It's crucial to make your boundaries known to your partner before you enter a committed relationship.

Girls are sensitive, feeling, kind, mature, and so forth. These are essentially the fundamental characteristics of a teenage girl. While in a relationship, they experience a wide range of emotions.

As they approach adolescence, they develop physically and become mentally quite confused by concepts like "love."

Teenage love feels completely insane. Setting boundaries would aid both parties in navigating their way through their relationship more successfully.

Boundaries can give adolescent girls a sense of security, relationship assurance, and control.

DATE WITHIN YOUR AGE-GROUP

The next and most crucial relationship advice I can give teenage girls is to date someone your own age.

I brought this up for two different reasons. The two of you will probably share common experiences and interests if you are dating a boy who is in your class or from a different school but is the same age as you.

Second, both parties will be at ease and understand each other.

Now, if you disagree, imagine that you are a teen girl dating a person who is seven years older than you. How likely is it that this relationship will endure or last long?

Even if it does, there will be a huge difference in the way that each of them thinks, as well as in their interests and points of view.

It would be preferable if you looked into dating or developing a deeper connection with someone your own age.

It's likely that your relationship will experience fewer difficulties and less negativity.

ONLY DATE WHEN YOU'RE SURE YOU'RE READY TO TAKE THAT STEP

All teenage girls are advised to only date or commit to a relationship when they are ready.

Teenage girls are weak both mentally and physically. They experience a great deal of change. These changes can sometimes befuddle them. They cannot set priorities. They constantly have a point to make.

For instance, you might feel the urge to date if you see that your best friend has a boyfriend. Even if you're not ready, you might start dating just to follow the trend and look hip.

It's important to take your time when it comes to dating and relationships. Before making any decisions about relationships because you are a teen girl, consult an adult who can mentor you and point you in the right direction.

Don't be too hard on yourself. Do not attempt it if you are not prepared. Await the appropriate moment and individual. Your heart will guide you if you follow.

DON'T RUSH INTO PHYSICAL INTIMACY

Teenage girls should be cautious when engaging in physical intimacy. Because of the hormones, physical desire is quite obvious.

Never be afraid to say "No" if your boyfriend asks you to engage in physical intimacy with him before you are ready.

It is crucial that both parties are fully aware of the risks associated with getting physical activity and how to engage in it safely.

It's best to first acquire the necessary knowledge if you are afraid.

Always keep in mind that you are only a teenager with plenty of time to explore. Therefore, take your time engaging in sexual activity.

AVOID DATING TOXIC INDIVIDUALS.

I would strongly advise waiting to find the right partner before you rush into a relationship.

In a toxic relationship, it is very challenging to remain alive, happy, and positive. You must have the patience to watch the behavior of the boys you are dating as a teen girl.

You are obviously old enough to judge a person. Ask your parents or older siblings for assistance. Always prefer waiting and watching than remaining in a toxic relationship.

During our teen years, I observed a few of my friends being emotionally blackmailed by their boyfriends and feeling trapped and stressed because of the toxic relationship they were in.

All teenage girls should exercise caution and, if they are already in a toxic relationship, dare to confide in someone who can offer them support.

DO NOT PUT YOUR RELATIONSHIP ON SOCIAL MEDIA

As you are aware, the internet is a web of shady practices. It serves as an endless playground for those who are looking for attention. Online predators can use your data and photos without your knowledge as well.

Numerous studies and research papers demonstrate how the internet takes advantage of adolescent boys and girls.

You are not required to post pictures or announce to the online community that you are dating if you are in a new relationship.

Keep your relationship off of social media and in private. Your relationship will avoid unneeded attention thanks to it.

Social media is not necessary if you and your partner are happy and content in your relationship.

DON'T BECOME OVERLY ATTACHED

Being in a relationship as a teenager feels good. You learn how to love someone selflessly and experience new feelings and emotions.

You are, however, suffocating both yourself and your partner in your relationship when that love becomes excessive.

Your emotional fragility will increase as you grow closer to your partner, and if the relationship ends, it will have a significant negative impact on you.

Can you handle heartache when you're a teenager?

I am aware that having too much invested in a relationship is unhealthy, especially for teenagers. There will be many ups and downs for you. When you are emotionally weak, managing yourself can be challenging.

Your overall well-being will be impacted by your mental health. Your academic performance, physical well-being, and interactions with other people will all be impacted.

Keep your relationship casual when you're a teen, it's one of my best relationship tips. Give your boyfriend some space, build trust, and enjoy yourself.

It's a really good idea to go on casual dates.

BE GRATEFUL TO ONE ANOTHER.

Teenage love is frequently observed to lack respect and appreciation for one another.

Keep in mind that gratitude is a strong emotion that can improve your relationship. Give your boyfriend the respect they deserve if you have one.

If your pocket money allows, you can express your gratitude with simple acts of kindness like writing a brief note of thanks or giving a thoughtful gift.

When it comes to boyfriends, teen girls can be sensible.

LOWER YOUR EXPECTATIONS.

You may be in love as an adolescent girl, which is wonderful. But if you want to be cautious and prevent yourself from getting wounded, keep your expectations in check.

You see, in a committed relationship, couples often have high expectations of one another. However, you shouldn't worry as much about meeting each other's expectations in a casual relationship.

The greatest method to inform one another of expectations is through effective communication. It will be simpler for both of you to maintain a sense of balance in your relationship the more open you are to discussing expectations.

For instance, if you expect your lover to remember every single detail about your likes and dislikes, you may discover him to be the complete opposite.

If you express your expectations to him clearly, you can avoid the argument that will inevitably result.

BE AUTHENTIC.

Teenage males and girls tend to value appearance above authenticity. Their perspectives of the outside world are extremely dissimilar. They believe that by being arrogant and pretentious, the other gender will find them attractive.

That is just incorrect.

Be creative if you want to strengthen and prolong your connection. When you are with your lover, be who you are. Let them know your good and bad characteristics. Allow them to accept you as you are.

Whether you're a male or a girl in your adolescent years, sincerity always prevails.

ALWAYS PROTECT YOURSELF

Teenage girls must possess a strong sense of self-awareness about their identities, rights, and how to defend themselves when around boys.

Teenage boys differ from one another. Some people lack empathy, don't understand how to respect women, have a conservative mindset, and treat their girlfriends brutally to keep them in check.

Studies consistently demonstrate the rise in teen relationships that are abusive. When one partner's thinking becomes oppressive, the dynamics of a relationship change. Some boys think they are strong and have control over women or girls.

Teenage girls need to know when to leave an abusive relationship and how to defend themselves from boyfriends.

Never forget to observe, comprehend, and evaluate a person before you do something.

BE PREPARED FOR HEARTBREAK

Heartbreaks in a relationship are inevitable. It won't always give you butterflies in your stomach if you're in love or dating someone. There will be hardships, obstacles, and heartbreaks as well.

Heartbreaks in relationships are the worst for teenagers, boys, and adults. Breakups will occur, so you'll need to learn how to handle them. You might also experience unrequited love, or one-sided love, to put it simply.

Teenage girls who are looking for relationship advice should know that they don't have to be prepared to experience heartbreak or feel afraid.

If something unplanned occurs, the experience will fortify you so that you can endure the suffering and heartbreak. Teenage girls are more responsible and mature than their male counterparts, and they are self-aware.

However, you shouldn't let that stop you from savoring the sensation of being in love.

NEVER FORGET YOUR STUDIES BECAUSE YOU'RE DATING.

Never skip classes while you are a teen girl dating or in a relationship. You can keep treating your studies seriously and push your partner to do the same.

Both will enroll in college to further their education after high school. You can use your free time to study with a friend. aspire to go on joint adventures after school.

I've known a lot of couples who were in long-lasting, fulfilling relationships before getting married. After meeting in high school, they remained together by encouraging one another's career and educational goals.

ALWAYS MAKE SURE YOU GET PRIORITY.

You are only a young woman. You don't have to give up anything or make concessions in your relationship. Now is the time to develop, learn, and enjoy yourself. It's unhealthy for you to continue being in a bad relationship and constantly put your boyfriend before yourself.

In the event that you are a teenage girl and have already adopted your boyfriend's lifestyle. At such a young age, you are engaged in risky behavior.

It may negatively impact your health and wellbeing.

Give up constantly attempting to make your partner happy. Consider yourself first. Being a little selfish is acceptable. You two are wed or have made a commitment to one another.

You are a teenage girl with a family and life that are separate from a boyfriend. Make yourself happy and act in your own best interests.

EMBRACE REJECTION WITH POSITIVITY.

For a teen, experiencing rejection in a relationship can be difficult. But this is only the beginning.

In some cases, despite your best efforts to make the relationship work, your significant other may not care as much about you or make you feel the way you do. It will undoubtedly hurt. Can you handle it?

Be mature enough to comprehend the reasons behind the rejection. Accept with grace and continue.

DON'T ALLOW YOUR BOYFRIEND TO CONTROL YOU.

If your boyfriend has a history of using deception and oppression, he might adore you, but he has the final say in your decisions and thoughts.

Think that's a good idea?

You can help yourself more effectively the sooner you realize it.

Talk to your boyfriend if you notice any problems with his controlling behavior. Better to move on if that situation doesn't change.

SPEND TIME DATING.

This is a crucial relationship advice I could offer if you are dating someone.

Don't rush into finding the right partner; instead, take your time. You're still a teen, so the dating scene is wide open. There is lots of time.

So go slowly and pay attention to the qualities of the guy you're dating. Recognize the qualities your ideal Mr. Right should possess and wait for the appropriate moment.

www.ingramcontent.com/pod-product-compliance
Lightning Source LLC
LaVergne TN
LVHW010216070526
838199LV00062B/4607